Useful tips
to become 120 years

Written by
Doctor Live Long

About the book

Doctor Live Long is very impressed by how an increasingly large group of people reach 100 years and more. According to different sources, many countries have a person living today at age 105-110. We are pretty sure there is a person at 115 living today, and we had one who reached 122 (and a half). There is even one man today who claims he is 145, but the evidence is not acceptable it seems.

Nevertheless, people are getting older than before, and there is no longer spectacular to turn 90. Life expectancy in developed countries is in fact soon reaching those 90 years. In a small country like Norway, with 5 million inhabitants, there will soon be 10 000 people alive who is 100 years or more. This gives hope for every individual who wants a long life.

At the same time, Doctor Long is not very satisfied with how the media present the recipe of reaching a high age. She feels that the average report from the sick bed is a man or woman turning 106, and the reporter ask: how did you get that old? The old jubilant then answers: I took a nap every day.

The intention behind this book is to present a nice selection of good advices for those who want to reach 120 years. There is no doubt that more and more people will accomplish this, and Long is convinced most of them will have followed many of the tips in this book (even without knowing the book exist).

Chapter 1: Genes

Tip number 1: Luck

Do you feel that you have good genes?
If your answer is yes, lucky you! Maybe your parents had good genes and passed them through to you. Maybe your mother chose a male with high probability to give her a healthy child. Good genes are a gift for you, a good foundation to achieve the goal of surviving many years. For you, the focus should be on picking the right life style to stay alive until you reach 120.
If your answer is no: It is impossible for you to choose your genes! You may think it's unfair that your friend or neighbor had more luck than you, but how will this help you to become 120? Your focus should be to disprove those who think you will die at 80. Adjust your life style to achieve your potential.

Tip number 2: Family history

There are many hereditary illnesses and diseases. Having one of them in your family can make you anxious, but your focus should be to discover as much fact as you can about the disease. Your mother said she had disease X. Is that proven, or did she just think it? Can you ask her to show you her medical history so that you can evaluate it yourself? What did she do to decrease the symptoms of that disease? Has medical science evolved since she was diagnosed? What is the probability to pass such a disease to a child? How can you live a life where you prevent that disease? As you understand, you have a detective's job to do, and you can only blame yourself if you choose not to do this necessary and important task.

Chapter 2: Nutrition (what you eat and drink)

Tip number 3: Eat more fish

Fish is the best source of omega-3, which is good both for your body and for your brain. Eating more fish will also give you a lot of vitamin D, a vitamin that prevents many diseases.
Fish is a universe of different tastes and recipes. Make sure you vary between all sorts of fish and seafood: salmon, trout, cod, halibut, shrimps, scampi, shells, etc.
When you travel to different countries, some people don't dear to try the local fish, but the fact is that the fish is often prepared safe and under high temperature, making it safe to eat. A good fish soup or bouillabaisse, a grilled local fish, these are often the best culinary surprises if you dear to try.
A fish meal often makes you feel more comfortable in your stomach compared to red meat, and it makes your digestive system work better.

Tip number 4: Eat more fruit and vegetables

5 times a day keeps your doctor away! It may seem like a lot, especially if you are not used to eating fruit and vegetables. The advice refers to portions of 100 grams, so it's not like you must eat 5 large items. To achieve this goal, it is evident to start in the grocery store. Make it a habit to buy the seasonal fruit and vegetables all times of the year, this will give you a good mix of proteins and a lot of fiber.

If you slice up some carrots and apples, it will be natural for you to use this as evening snacks, instead of less healthy alternatives.

Cut down on the meat, 150 grams can make you just as happy as 250 grams. Focus more on how you prepare those 150 grams, make the beef tender and combine with fresh vegetables.

Tip number 5: Eat your food rawer

Did you know that a medium rare steak is healthier than a well-done steak? Your body will use more energy to digest the rawer steak, making the calorie balance more favorable.

Do not just press out the juice and throw away the fruit meat! This will give you the sugar of the fruit, but not the fibers. Eat it as raw as you can, and let it be a natural part of the meals.

Use lower temperature and longer time when you prepare food. Instead of overcooking it, you will control the heating process and stop it at the best time.

Tip number 6: Eat more fiber

A lot of people have problems with their digestive system. Eating more fiber-rich food will make your intestine function better, and it will prevent constipation and other stomach related illnesses. There are many health benefits associated with a fiber-rich diet: it will make it easier for you to go to the toilet regularly since your stool will be more soft and easier to get out. Your cholesterol will go down. Your blood sugar level will be better. It will be easier for you to control your weight.

Fiber is essential, just try it! You can start by eating more whole wheat bread, and more crispbread.

Tip number 7: Cut down on sugar

Animals don't have much sugar in their natural diet, nor did humans. Sugar was introduced as a cheap ingredient which also have an addiction effect on people. When the world's largest Champagne producer have a special edition for Americans, a Champagne with more sugar added, you start to understand the sugar addiction.
Don't be fanatic, just replace sugar intensive groceries with less sugar intensive alternatives. Coke zero instead of regular coke. Use less sugar in cakes. Eat more fruit sugar instead of added sugar. Make it a gradually transition, this will increase your success rate.
Sugar is not dangerous for you if you limit the amount you eat. If you eat too much, it will be stored in your body as fat, and you might be overweight. This again can lead to diabetes.

Tip number 8: Reduce salt

The more salt you eat, the higher blood pressure you get. This can lead to heart attack, strokes and other related illnesses. Most processed food you buy at grocery stores have too much salt added, to ensure a good taste.
The food industry has started to act by gradually reducing the amount of salt added. This process goes too slowly, therefore you should try to make food from natural ingredients instead of buying processed food. If you do that you can control the amount of salt added, and you can use other things to enhance taste, such as ginger, garlic, lemon, chili and herbs.
The same problem happens in restaurants, the chefs add a lot of salt to ensure that you taste a lot, and many guests add even more salt, often by habit.
Try to gradually add less salt on your food, eventually it will taste just as good as before, with less salt added.

Tip 9: Eat less fat

To control your cholesterol level, you should reduce the
amount of fat in your diet. The easiest way is to reduce visible
fat such as fatty parts of your steak, sausages, cream, ice-
cream, butter, oil, margarine, cheese, fried food. Most
processed food also contains a lot of fat, such as pastries,
cookies, and cakes. Make it a habit to have healthier
alternatives available in your home, so that you easily can eat
a fruit between meals, instead of a cookie.
If the fat lays around your waist, you are in significant danger
of getting a heart disease and to develop type 2 diabetes.
If you want to become 120 years old, you must eat less fat.

Chapter 3: Eating behaviour

Tip 10: Eat small portions often.

Have you heard about this research with rats: some rats got small portions and was a little hungry all the time, while others could eat more? The hungry ones lived longer.

Sounds boring to be hungry, right?
The point is that you should not eat heavy meals twice a day, instead you should eat small portions often. In that way your stomach will be smaller, since it doesn't have to store food for many hours. Try to adjust your intake so that you have a more even flow of food through your system. You may experience that you enjoy it more, and you will for sure avoid those moments in the sofa where you feel so stuffed that you lack energy to do any activities. As for all changes in diets: do it gradually and evaluate constantly.

Tip 11: Eat varied

If you eat smaller portions, you can also eat unhealthy food with better conscience, since you then only eat small portions of that less healthy food/snack.
A varied diet will ensure that your body receives necessary vitamins and minerals. It will increase illness immunity, ensure a good development and better healing of the body, increase energy so that you can do more activities, improve your concentration etc.
A varied diet will prevent a vast number of diseases and increase the ability to live long. When you get older, this variation can preserve your appetite and your joy of living.

Tip 12: Eat slowly

If you eat more slowly, you will digest your food easier, and your toilet routines can improve. Eating slowly can help you to maintain a healthy weight. It can also help you to enjoy your meals more by focusing on the different ingredients. Your hydration will be better, and you will also feel fuller before you have loaded the extra portion on your plate, making you control your intake better.

The meal experience can also be better if you focus more on the persons you share the meal with. Take small breaks during the meal to prolong the experience.

Tip 13: Keep your appetite at high age

Focusing on how you eat, what you eat, and who you eat with, can give you better appetite at all ages, but particularly when you turn 90 and 100. Too many old people stop eating and die much earlier than necessary. It is highly important to find joy in food even when you come to a nursing home.

At such high ages, it may be good to loosen a bit on your strictest rules, since most people get too thin when they turn 100. Make food your new hobby and spend some more money on it than you previously did. Give your body a boost so that you live those extra 10 years.

Tip 14: Avoid obesity

You probably know that obesity leads to increased risk of numerous diseases and illnesses? Your heart must work harder to pump out blood to a larger body, and this could lead to higher blood pressure, heart diseases and stroke. The risk of getting diabetes increases if you are heavily overweighted. You can get breathing problems such as sleep apnea and asthma. Several organs, such as your liver and kidneys, will get problems earlier than necessary. Your self-esteem goes down, and your enjoyment of life decreases.

The solution is to eat less. Start by reducing the amount of food slowly by eating 5 % smaller meals. Your stomach will adapt to this so that you gradually get satisfied with a decreased intake of calories. Continue this process if you feel comfortable or if you want to reduce weight. Before you try any "magic" diets, eat the same as before, but a little bit less than before. Start by reducing the amount you put on the plate. If you are eating from a buffet, plan to go several times instead of putting it all on one plate.
Obesity will make you die younger than necessary.

Chapter 4: Exercise

Tip 15: The everyday training

Did you know that 2/3 of the daily calorie burning is done by simply existing? Your body needs energy to do normal body functions like breathing, pumping blood, digesting etc. This mean that you only need to focus on the remaining 1/3, good news, right?
Several studies now show that it is the everyday training that is the most important source of burning calories. Everyday training means that you try to stay active during a large part of the day. Make sure you walk those extra metres when you go to work, taking the stairs instead of the elevator, choosing the second nearest bus stop, raise up and walk around in your office, do small errands. When you come home, do some housework or some gardening, walk the dog, play with your kids, visit your neighbour. All these small things add up to significant calorie burning and improves your body machinery.

Tip 16: Do some organized activity

Being part of some organized activity will give you structure in your exercise. Having 1-3 weekly appointments will make it more likely for you to attend at least some of them. Don't be so strict that you cannot cancel if you get other plans, but make sure you are a part of a group where others encourage you to show up and share the same interest as you. Don't exaggerate, top athletes don't necessarily live a healthy life. One of the reasons why people only live 80 years is that they quit organized activity just because they are "over the top". Simply adjust your activities to your age and how fit you are.

Tip 17: Strengthen your muscles

Doing some strength and weight training gives numerous positive effects on your body, and the importance increases as older you become. Make sure you have some weight manuals available for ad hoc training. Do some push ups, sit ups, squats on a regular basis. Remember that muscles need to be used to function properly. Strength is not something you reach when you are young and stays with you till you die! Strength is something fresh that constantly needs to be maintained. Some light weight training is perfect for reducing inflammations and strain injury. Building strength is evident when you get older and need to recover after a broken bone or an operation. Muscles give you some extra years!
And listen: you feel wonderful after some minutes of muscles training.

Tip 18: Reduce medication

A drug sometimes saves lives and make you feel better.
But, we are now overusing medicine in most countries, leading to dangerous side effects and antibiotic resistance. Too many people take pills and medicine to reduce pain, instead of going to the root of the problem.
Try to find the origin of your problem and fix it yourself. Stretching, back exercises, alternative training when you're injured, mobility training, stress release, breathing exercises. Exercise is a pain killer for your back, shoulders, knees, hips. Go for a walk and sleep better after. Common sense is often the best medication.

Tip 19: Strengthen your heart

Endurance training is the act of performing a task over time,
such as jogging, cycling, swimming, cross country skiing.
When you get older: walking with some speed, uphill
walking, climbing some stairs. The important thing for you is
to adjust the effort so that you get higher pulse and train your
heart so that you strengthen/remain endurance, even at high
age. Training your heart gives you lower every day pulse, the
heart doesn't have to beat so many times to give you a good
blood stream. This will make your heart rest better. Typical
can a well-trained athlete have 40 heart beats per minute
when he (woman often a bit higher) rest, while a non-trained
person can have 80. This is a significant difference, and the
non-trained person will die sooner.

Also remember that the heart is a muscle, and muscle strength
is something you need to keep "fresh". This means you
should never stop training endurance. Imagine you get in a
situation where something scares you, or maybe you need to
react quick on a danger, you will want to have a heart that is
used to pulse changes so that you don't get a heart attack.
One quick advice: do not go for not-trained to hard training,
this could be dangerous. Take it in your own tempo, and listen
to your heart, do not overdo it.

Chapter 5: Modern medicine

Tip 20: Listen to your body

Many illnesses and diseases give you a warning before it's too
late. You have probably heard about a father or grandfather
who suddenly fell to the ground because of heart problems.
Typically, they overdid some work task (snow shovelling,
digging a ditch, etc). In recent past, very few persons were
able to listen to the early signals from their body. You should
learn how to examine yourself, and to interpret signals.
During an exercise or work performance, pain in a body part
can be an early sign that tells you to stop the movement. In the
long run, it is better for you to reduce the stress on that muscle
instead of having to rebuild it completely later.
Changes in your skin or in your health can be early signals of
a disease or an illness.
To many waits for years before they dear to ask for a
professional view. When there is something abnormal with
you, go to the doctor!

Tip 21: Avoid cancer

Many types of cancer can be avoided by examining yourself.
Testicular cancer and breast cancer can often be avoided by
thoroughly examination by simply using your hands during a
shower. You don't even need to know what you are looking
for, just get familiar with how the body feels, and watch out
for changes. Typically, there could be a lump in your
breast/testicle, pain or discomfort. If it lasts for a while,
discuss it with your doctor.

You can reduce the risk of getting lung cancer by not smoking.
This is the easiest tip to avoid cancer. You know what to do.

Other tips to reduce cancer: Eat food from plant sources, avoid obesity, be careful with strong sun, check your skin often for irregularities. The best advice is to go to the doctor regularly and discuss cancer risk. Even doctor Google can help you with this.

Tip 22: Reduce stress

Stress gives you heart problems, right? Or not?
There are numerous studies about stress. Some of them gives an indirect link between stress and heart problems, by stating that if you feel stressed, you tend to behave unhealthy by eating wrong, exercising to little etc, hence increasing the probability that you will get heart problems. Others focus on the direct link, for example that high level of stress can give an unfortunate blood flow through your body, causing blood clots. Stress in a certain moment can give you a heart attack. No matter how you look at it, it is good to invest in a stress-free environment, and to be aware of when you typically get stressed, so that you can avoid it.

Tip 23: Digestion

Poor digestion can be critical for your body. Bad food can give you bacteria imbalance in your gut and bowel. A good diet of healthy food, including a lot of fiber, will help you to have a good balance in your digestion. Some people drink so little fluid that they get problems with pooping. This is very serious, and unnecessary if you have clean water available. Good digestion is very much linked with nutrition, exercise and good mental health. The good thing is that your visits at the toilet will tell you whether you are in balance or not. Monitor irregularities: how often do you pee? How often do you poop? How is the colour? How is the texture? Is there any blood in your urine or in your poop? How does your stomach feel? When you notice irregularities, be analytic and think about what you have eaten lately, whether you have exercised lately, etc. Be your own digestion consultant!

Tip 24: Operations

Many people get a new chance to live long by getting operated for an illness. Your focus should be to discover your personal need for an operation, early. By monitoring your body functions, going do the doctor, listening to signs, you can early discover challenges that need to be addressed. It is no shame to get an operation if one of your organs need to be repaired or even replaced. Doing an operation when you still got the strength to go through with it, can give you the necessary help to maintain a healthy life, with the life style needed to reach a high age.

Tip 25: The next cure

Modern medicine has developed in an impressive speed over the last years, and it seems like it will continue even faster. Maybe the next cure will be the one that help you to become 120 years old. Your focus should be on two things: monitoring the development within the cures that you are most likely to need in the future and planning how you can afford it when needed.

Chapter 6: Mental health

Tip 26: Anger management

Many people get angrier when they age. They feel that the world has gone against them, and their lives didn't turn out as expected. If you don't find a way to manage this kind of anger, it can really be negative for your mental health. The bitterness and feeling of injustice can be a negative spiral that make it hard to gain and maintain friends, and it may lead to an unhappy life. Sometimes it can help with some simple techniques to control your temper (think before you speak, count to 10, relax, take a deep breath). Frequent exercise can help you to drain out some of the negative feelings. If you notice that you have a serious problem with your anger, you should seek help from professionals.

Tip 27: Positive thinking

It is very easy to focus on some sad things from the past, or some problems that made your life more difficult. Traditionally, many people in their 50's start to look back on their life instead of ahead. Focusing on the future instead of the past will make you see opportunities. If you want to live 120 years, why should you stop making long term plans when you are 60? Why should you stop exercising when you are 80? Positive thinking is a difficult task, especially if you are in the middle of some serious problems. Doctor Live Long emphasise that this skill is something you must develop over time, by constantly reminding you how fortunate you are to be alive, and how special you are as a unique human being.

Tip 28: Accepting change

If you become 100, 110, 120 years old, you must have experienced a lot of change during your life. You can see a huge difference among today's seniors. Some of them have embraced new technology and smart solutions. Others have cursed all change because they hate to adopt to new routines. Accepting that the younger generation decides the world's direction is probably the most important choice to make. Being curious on new technology, new food and drinks, trying new medias, talking to new people, all of this can make it easier to live a long life.

Tip 29: Forgiveness

After living a long life, people tend to regret all the times they were angry on someone, situations where they were too strict on following some principles. You eventually understand that life is not black/white, both parts are responsible for how it turned out. Typically, you can be angry because you didn't get enough love and attention from family members, a near friend stood you up, a relationship ended badly, a boss fired you. Such feelings seldom help you to have a healthy mind. If you develop the skill of forgiveness early in life, you may find that it enriches your life by giving you more friends, more family around you, and a lighter mind. All of this will help you to reach a high age.

Tip 30: Family and friends

Typically, humans that live very long have lost many family members and friends. Either they have died earlier than you, or you have lost contact with them. Most people focus on getting friends when they are 20-30, and family when they are 30-40. If you are to become 120 years old, you must shift your focus and make it a whole-life strategy. This means that some of us will need to build a new family, others will closely follow up great grandchildren. Others again focus more on constantly getting new friends by participating in activities where you meet new people. Having social setting in your life will improve your feeling of happiness and will prolong your life.

Tip 31: Love and sex

All you need is love.
Well, that's not true, but love is something that make your life better, and therefore increases your age expectancy. Love does not have to be the ONE love in your life, it can simply be the good feeling you have towards a partner, your family, your friends, your pet. If you can give love, it is more likely that you receive love. Love is one of the few things that doesn't diminish when you give it to someone.
If you are in your mid ages (60-70) it is very well possible that you have lost one you loved. You must dear to love again! Remember that you have many decades left, and you would like to have more love in your life.

Tip 32: Nature

Nature is a miracle cure. Staying near a park, a river, a lake, a hiking track, the forest…using the nature for recreation…you must try it to understand it. There are many religions in the world, but no one can argue against the power of nature, how plants and trees and flowers go through the different seasons of the year. Many people, especially elders, find peace and happiness by spending time in nature. This give you good mental health and strengthen your ability to avoid mental illnesses. It is also very much likely to give you more exercise, which will contribute to a long and healthy life.

Tip 33: Curiosity

It is important to maintain the joy of life. For many people, life becomes boring with routines repeating themselves week after week, year after year. Some people lose the ability to be curious on things, failing to get new hobbies, not getting new friends, being sceptic about new things and new people, instead of being interested and curious, eager to learn something new. Instead you should look at children how they approach the world and try to maintain the little child inside of you. Life has enormous amounts of areas to study, things to learn. Stay curious!

Tip 34: Pets

Pets are fun to play with, and they can give you exercise. Owning a pet can also reduce depression, lower your blood pressure, and reduce probability of heart diseases. It can be worth it to have this in mind when you plan your 80's or your 90's. You may not want to have a dog on your own, but maybe you can share one with your neighbor or someone in your family? Pets also tend to give you extra exercise, either by walking a dog or by playing with your cat.

Tip 35: Humor

Laugh a lot, choose situations where it's more likely you will find something funny. Choose the friends you find amusing, watch comedies online, go to stand up shows etc. Take a glass of wine and watch an extra episode of that funny YouTube moment. Just make sure you laugh! Laughter can give you many health benefits, such as reduce stress, lower blood pressure, release endorphins, making you feel well, making your body relax, helps the immune system, protects the heart, burn calories. Laughter makes your mental health better by reducing anxiety and by general improvement of your mood. It can also help you to get new friends, to maintain relations, and to avoid conflicts. All this will prolong your life.

Tip 36: Reducing anxiety

Some people are born with more anxiety than others. It can be very hard, even impossible, to remove anxiety. The best choice would be to learn how to live with it. First step is to accept that you are an anxious person. Most people understand intellectually that they are more anxious than they need to be, but the brain still make you feel afraid or anxious. By recognising the areas and moments that makes you most anxious, you can learn to cope with it. It is seldom a good idea to sit quiet and focus on the anxiety, the better solution is to think: what happened last time I did something like this? It went well, even though I was anxious. I must try to go through with this task one more time. After you have done it, take a moment and tell you: it went well this time as well!

Tip 37: Choose your friends

Some people take away your energy instead of giving you joy. The most challenging ones are those with personality disorders. These are the ones that constantly conflict with their surroundings, including their so-called friends (you). It could be worth it to spot these persons early in a relationship and choose not to spend much time with them. There are many types of abnormal behavior, these are examples:
-   The one who only think about their ego and doesn't really listen to you or respect you as an equal person
-   The one who constantly shifts between being incredible happy (I love you) and bottomless sad/angry (I hate you)
-   The one who want to give you bad conscience for everything
-   The one who doesn't support you when you are in a tough period

Choose to spend time with people who give you good energy, and if you have some energy to share, help one who need that extra energy.

Chapter 7: Avoiding risk behavior

Tip 38: Accidents

Risk behavior leads to more accidents. It is not hard to understand why more men than women are killed in car accidents, they have a higher likeliness to drive faster and to take risks in the traffic. Other typical risky things to do: being to near moving machinery, not looking out for falling objects, falling hard on slippery surfaces, trying to repair something in the ceiling or at the roof with not enough security measures. Many of these accidents can be avoided by being aware of the possible dangers involved in activities, and to actively thinking about how you can reduce them. It is very important to accept your limitations as you get older and older, you cannot do the same as before, it can be well worth it to pay someone to help you.

Tip 39: Railings and other equipment

Remember to always use railings when you climb stairs. Accidents by falling and breaking some bones can be the start of your final years. Typically, the surface will be very hard if you fall in stairs, in steep hills, or on winter ice roads. Recovering after a broken bone or an injured hip gets harder as older you get. It is therefore important that you focus on using equipment that prevents you from falling: canes, crampons, good shoes, relevant tools, safety lines etc.

Choosing not to use recommended equipment is risk behavior that will shorten your life.

Tip 40: Suicide

Some say that the number of people dying by suicide is approximately the same as the number dying by car accidents. The figure is around 1.4 % of all deaths. The older you get, the more difficult it is to notice all suicides. Some people get tired of living and disguise their suicide as a "normal" death. The first times you get suicidal thoughts, take them seriously! Try to understand why you are tired of life and try to do something with it. Seek professional help if needed. There are many ways to get help, you can start by trying to find a phone number to organizations who has hotlines where you can talk with a person about your problems.

Tip 41: Retirement

Finally, I can retire…I don't have to do anything…

This is a very risky approach. Of course, you deserve to retire, but are you sure you want to do it now? If you plan to be 120, how many years are left now? Should you try to work 5 more years?

Sometimes it's good to retire, if you find something useful to do, a hobby you can focus on, or some charity work for the community. Retirement only to rest, well, that is the beginning of your final sleep. Find the interesting tasks that will keep you going those extra years.

Tip 42: Alcohol abuse

The information about the danger of abusing alcohol is very much available for the public. Why do we still consume these dangerous products? The answer is probably that it gives you a sense of joy, relief, well-being. All though some research show that a glass of wine or two per day can have a good effect on your heart, there are several reasons why the authorities refuse to recommend you drink alcohol every day. One of the reasons is that alcohol can increase the risk of cancer. Alcohol is also very addictive, if you start to drink two glasses per day, it can easily be more, and the positive effect of your heart is lower than the negative effects on your body.

Tip 43: Drug abuse

This is a no brainer: do not use drugs. They will make you addictive, you will use more and more, and they will destroy your body and make you die younger than necessary.

Do not try it!

If you have tried it, stop using it!

Tip 44: Cigarettes and snuff

Why do people smoke? The nicotine quickly spreads via the lungs into the blood and gives you a pleasant feeling. Many uses it to avoid stress and distract negative feelings. Nicotine is one of the most addictive substances found in everyday life of people. It is charmless, smelly, and untrendy. It also cost a fortune that could have been used on better nutrition. And: it gives you cancer and make you die younger than necessary.

Do not use cigarettes or snuff!

Tip 45: Balance

You have probably heard of "the golden mean".

It states that if you don't overdo things, most thing are ok. Eat what you want, but not too much of the same thing. Eat a lot if you want but adjust your exercise to your intake. Enjoy some wine, but not a bottle every day. Harmony and balance should be your goal, not being extreme in any way. Try to see the whole picture in your life, try to figure out how the different parts of your life is linked together. Remember that your balance is not the same as others balance. If you succeed in finding the balance in your life, you will live longer.

Tip 46: Choose your 5 favorite tips

Hopefully you found some interesting tips in this book. Each one invites you to dig deeper into the subject. The last advice is to read the tips once more to get a better overview of the total thinking. You will probably find some of them obvious, others irrelevant. Discuss them with your friends. Choose a few tips where you have improvement potential, and work with these.

Good luck to you all!

Doctor Live Long anno 2019:

Doctor Live Long is 102 years old, and still going strong. She drinks a glass of wine every day and enjoy life.
Her focus now is to be a good conversation partner for some of her neighbours who are 80-101 years old. Her exercise consists of going for a walk every morning and every afternoon, the length of the walk is decided by how she feels that day. Once a day she picks up some training manuals and do some muscle training. She eats varied and invest some extra money in good food.

Maybe she is a little bit anxious about getting into an accident. Well, she can live with that.

18 years to go…